Enhanced *Beauty*

MEN'S GROOMING

*by Daytime Emmy Award-Winning Hairstylist
and Nominated Make-Up Artist*

D'ANGELO THOMPSON

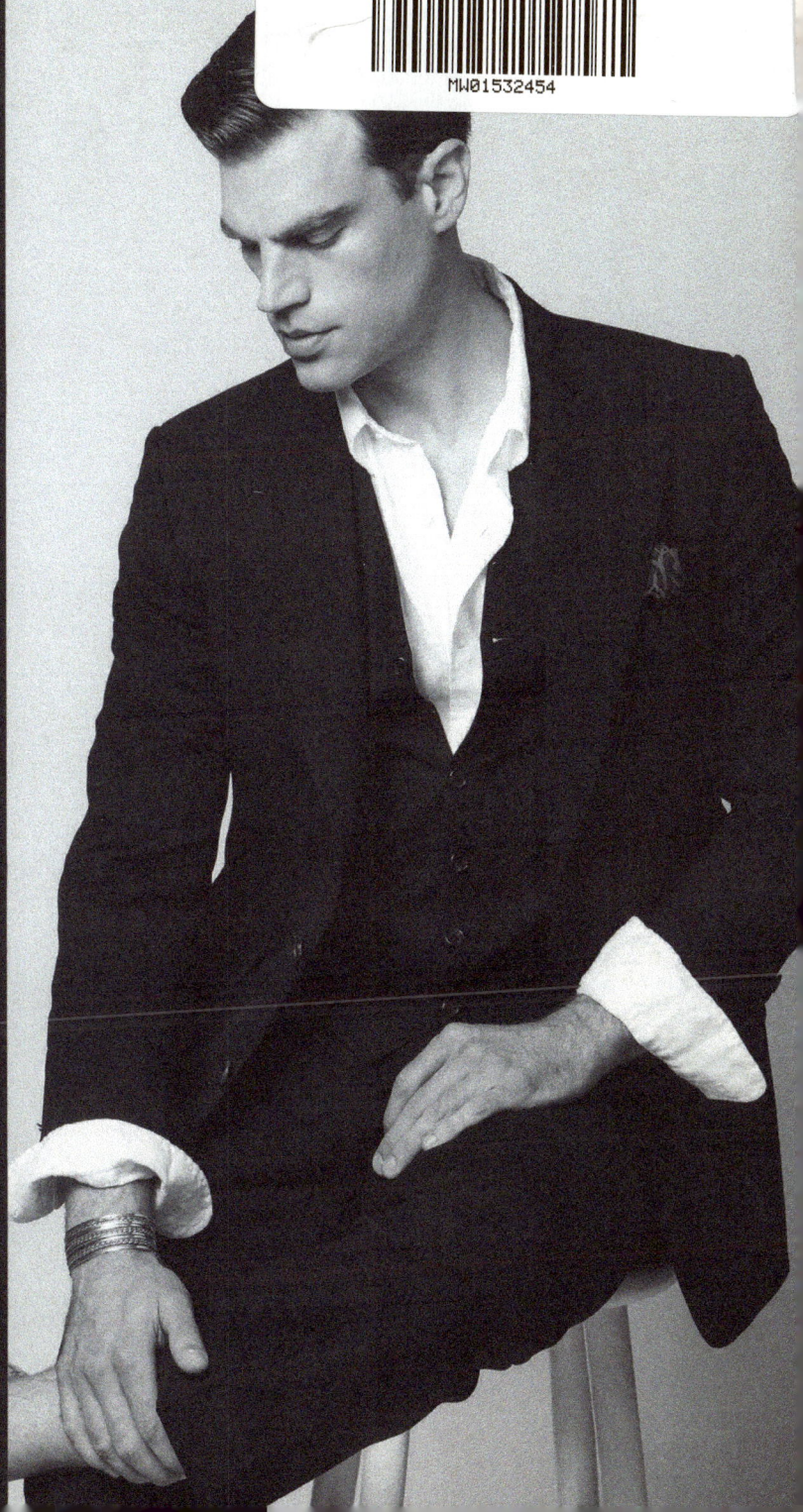

AuthorHouse™
1663 Liberty Drive
Bloomington, IN 47403
www.authorhouse.com
Phone: 1 (800) 839-8640

Published by AuthorHouse 12/07/2018

ISBN: 978-1-5462-6583-2 (sc)
ISBN: 978-1-5462-6582-5 (e)

Library of Congress Control Number: 2018912795

Print information available on the last page.

This book is printed on acid-free paper.

authorHOUSE

Enhanced *Beauty*

CREDITS:

PHOTOS/BTS IMAGES:	JASON ROTH
PORTRAIT PHOTO OF D'ANGELO:	ELIZABETH YOUNG
BACKCOVER PHOTO:	JUSTIN CLYNES
FORWARD:	D'ANGELO THOMPSON
PRODUCTION COORDINATOR:	EWA PERRY
GRAPHIC & LAYOUT DESIGN	FRITZ COLINET FROM RETNAMEDIA.COM
HAIR STYLISTS:	DENINE SMITH & D'ANGELO THOMPSON
HAIR TIPS:	DENINE SMITH, RAUL DA LUZ, MARCO GUGLIELMINO & DAVE RAKMAN
GROOMER:	D'ANGELO THOMPSON
EDITOR:	ADRIENNE PACE
FASHION STYLING/COVER:	D'ANGELO THOMPSON & DAVID CHIN
COVER MODEL:	PAUL KOCH
MODELS:	DR. CRAIG ZEBUDA, STEVEN DELVALLE, DAVID CHIN, JASON CHIN, DR. REGINALD GAY, CALVERT JOSEPH, EUGENE FLOTTERON, JADON FLOTTERON, DARREN FLOTTERON & DENNIS HOWARD

A VERY SPECIAL THANKS TO TERI FERGUSON-ROTH

"KNOWING YOURSELF IS THE BEGINNING OF ALL WISDOM."

- ARISTOTLE

Carmen & Marcos

Thank you for all your
support and kindness. I
appreciate you and enjoy
the book!!

Always invite the
energy of love, prosperity
and light into all aspects
of your life.
XOXO,
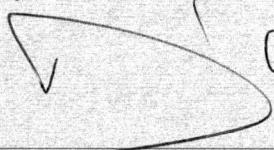
2019

FROM THE AUTHOR

T his book is dedicated to the men who inspire me daily and most importantly, my maternal grandfather, **Malachi Thompson**. I learned from the stories told to me that he was a very dapper and hard working man. Unfortunately, he lived a very short life in rural Mississippi after a work accident paralyzed him and I never got the opportunity to meet him. His legacy lives on through me, his eldest grandson, as well as through his daughter, three sons, grandchildren, great grandchildren and eventually his great, great grandchildren. Because of Malachi Thompson and many more before him, I strive to follow in his footsteps everyday by walking with honor, integrity, and class. He was the epitome of what I believe a gentleman to be.

D'angelo Thompson

Author, Beauty Entrepreneur and Make-Up Artist/Groomer

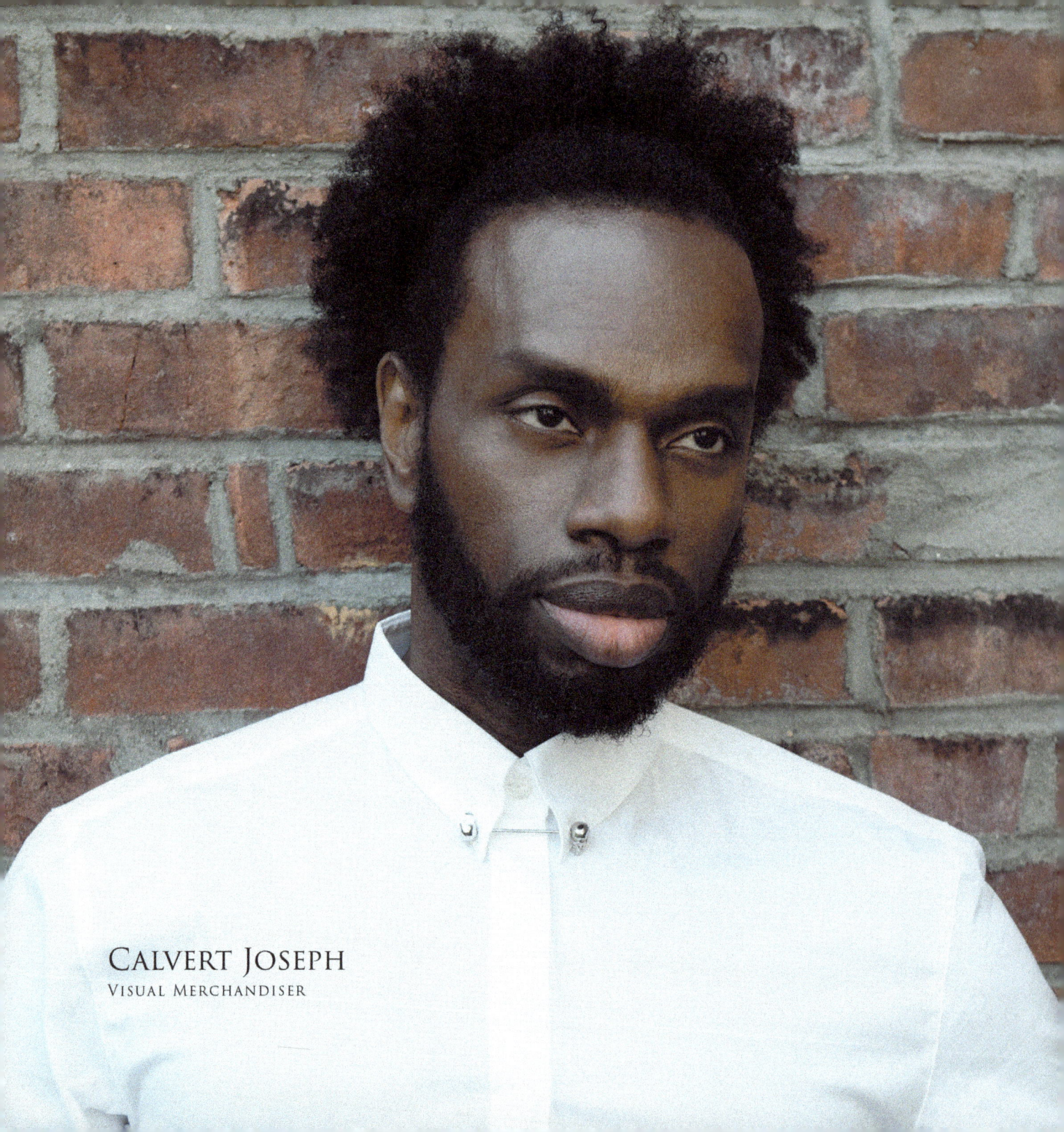

CALVERT JOSEPH
Visual Merchandiser

Calvert Joseph, a friend for over two decades, is not only a dear friend & brother, but also a loan officer, counselor and a man with exemplary fashion style; he has a flare for mixing all of the right fashion items together. He and David Chin are my go-to friends' when I need style advice for an event or when I want to add an item to my wardrobe.

Calvert has worked with many noted national and global accessory, fashion and home brands in visual merchandising, as well as a stylist on a multitude of photo shoots. Working as a visual merchandiser is a well-chosen career for him.

We met in 1989 as freshmen at Pratt Institute in the lobby of Pantos Dormitory. We gave each other the "once over" and made quick judgements. I knew I loved his complexion, European style and dared him to flirt with someone I was attracted to. Needless to say, what flourished was a long and honorable friendship.

When I enter Calvert's closet at his home in Harlem, I salivate at the wonderful designer pieces he has been able to keep and archive in optimal condition.

I am very thankful (he does not enjoy being photographed) that he graciously allowed us to photograph him, as well as take over his home for three hours.

So, this book is a tribute to my dear friend, Calvert, and men like him that are style icons everyday in their personal and professional lives.

Whether you believe in creation or are an evolutionist, one thing is certain -- the human species/man has come a very long way. From the very hairy, cave/tree dwelling primates like Lucy, who is the mother of us all, to Millennials. From the Neanderthal to the modern day Homo-sapiens ("metrosexuals" as we know them today)...humans have evolved tremendously.

Did you know that most human babies are covered with hair called "lanugo" while in their mother's womb and it starts to fall off the closer the baby comes to full term? I find this fact to be fascinating. It has made me think about how far we've come as a species geographically, mentally, spiritually and technologically, but yet, we are still connected to that primal part of our beginning.

Regardless of the millenniums that humans have inhabited this planet, the topic of grooming, especially male grooming, is still very perplexing to many.

Men's grooming is chronicled throughout history, especially in African, Asian, Latino, Native and Western cultures. If you dig a little deeper you can explore the male aesthetic throughout the world, mainly through cave drawings, carvings, etchings, oral history, art, literature, photography or by researching tribal or royal archives. The Museum of Natural History (NYC), The Metropolitan Museum of Art (NYC), The British Museum (London, England) or The Smithsonian Institute (Washington, D.C.) exhibitions and archives provide you a vast sampling of man's evolution.

In modern times men's grooming has been chronicled in men's quarterlies, print, film, television and digital fashion magazines. *The Great Gatsby* by F. Scott Fitzgerald is a great example of the care men took to look fashionable. Baz Luhrmann's production of the movie serves as the perfect example.

Did you know that barbers not only took care of men's grooming, but they were also known for

Whether you believe in creation or are an evolutionist, one thing is certain -- the human species/man has come a very long way. From the very hairy, cave/tree dwelling primates like Lucy, who is the mother of us all, to Millennials. From the Neanderthal to the modern day Homo-sapiens ("metrosexuals" as we know them today)...humans have evolved tremendously.

Did you know that most human babies are covered with hair called "lanugo" while in their mother's womb and it starts to fall off the closer the baby comes to full term? I find this fact to be fascinating. It has made me think about how far we've come as a species geographically, mentally, spiritually and technologically, but yet, we are still connected to that primal part of our beginning.

Regardless of the millenniums that humans have inhabited this planet, the topic of grooming, especially male grooming, is still very perplexing to many.

Men's grooming is chronicled throughout history, especially in African, Asian, Latino, Native and Western cultures. If you dig a little deeper you can explore the male aesthetic throughout the world, mainly through cave drawings, carvings, etchings, oral history, art, literature, photography or by researching tribal or royal archives. The Museum of Natural History (NYC), The Metropolitan Museum of Art (NYC), The British Museum (London, England) or The Smithsonian Institute (Washington, D.C.) exhibitions and archives provide you a vast sampling of man's evolution.

In modern times men's grooming has been chronicled in men's quarterlies, print, film, television and digital fashion magazines. *The Great Gatsby* by F. Scott Fitzgerald is a great example of the care men took to look fashionable. Baz Luhrmann's production of the movie serves as the perfect example.

Did you know that barbers not only took care of men's grooming, but they were also known for performing surgeries, which included bloodletting and dentistry? This is according to online sources like Wikipedia. There are references and historical barber relics found as far back as the Bronze Age in Egypt, as well as in Greece, who later introduced barbering to the Romans. The baths, which we now call spas or barbershops, are places where men from all backgrounds gather to discuss family and work, as well as political and social issues. Anyone who has sat in a barbershop or men's grooming salon could listen to or chime in on a variety of topics.

My main focus for this project is about mens grooming for the modern man to help men navigate choosing the right skincare, shaving products, hair products, barber cuts and or hair styling, body care/hygiene and overall wellness.

I spoke to many friends, colleagues and influencers about the topic of men's grooming tips as well as my own personal/professional experiences and anecdotes learned over two decades in an ever evolving profession. Hopefully this book will leave you with a wealth of useful tips and information.

As a young boy and through my teen years I didn't have much facial or body hair. I was always curious about shaving and couldn't wait to do it. I watched my uncles while they shaved. And sometimes my stepdad would let me watch his shaving process. He and his brother have great skin, so they never dealt with ingrown hairs.

However, all three of my maternal uncles had issues with ingrown hairs and acne as young men, especially my mother's middle brother. As I started to shave I had the same issue, which I will share with you in the next chapter and throughout the book.

SKINCARE

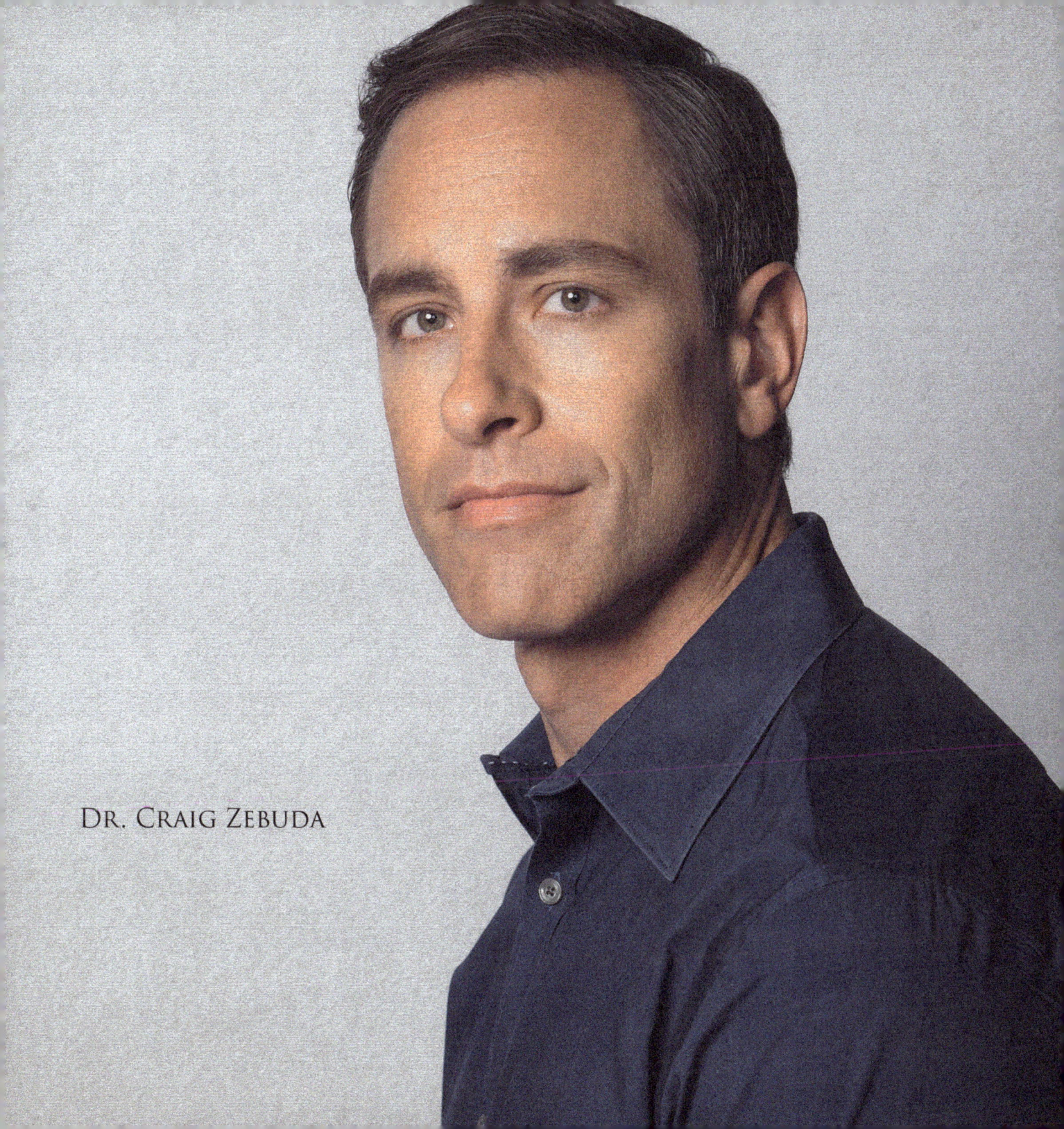

DR. CRAIG ZEBUDA

Some people are born with great skin. My buddy, Dr. Craig Zebuda, takes pride in his appearance. This is clearly demonstrated in his commitment to fitness and the care he takes with grooming. A lot of men have to work at having great skin. Craig does not.

Puberty for most boys sends our hormones and skin into unwanted distress from ages 9-14, as per kidshealth.org During this stage some boys/teens start to have acne, ingrown hairs and/or other skin issues that can last into their early 20's. It's important to get a jumpstart on what the best skincare regimen is for your particular skin. Deep cleansing, hydrating and moisturizing the skin will help to regulate and get rid of acne-causing bacteria. Also, some skin issues stem from your diet, genetics or the environment, so it's good to be conscious about the foods you choose in your diet. Wearing SPF is paramount for skin protection. Sun Protection Factor (SPF) prevents acne scars from getting darker, as well as protects against UVA/UVB rays. It can also leave the skin looking more evened out, especially after sun exposure.

I know as young boys you don't always have the power of whats being fed to you daily but most teens and adults are very specific with their food needs and or likes. Its a great conversation you can approach with your parents about healthier food options or even planting a garden together. I actually had many gardens ages between 7-12 years old while growing up in rural Mississippi. I enjoyed watching things grow and being able to cook a meal from your own garden is priceless and yes i could cook a decent meal by age ten. I would goto country general stores to buy seeds or order from the back of my grandmother's catalogs to buy seeds that were like 10 cents and plant them and VOILA fresh tomatoes, melons and even beans months later.

One thing you do have control over is how you take care of your face and body. Being active and focusing on hygiene are important steps to having great skin and maintaining your health down the road.

There are hundreds of brands on the market that cater to male and female consumers for skincare and skin protection, but for the sake of this book I'll focus on skincare products for men. Take a stroll in any pharmacy anywhere in the world, a beauty floor in a department store and the skincare section of your favorite organic food store or spa. There's always something for you. Even as close to you as your kitchen there are items in the cupboard or fridge that will help your skin look and feel better.

The one thing that's helped mens' skin for centuries is shaving. It's a way of deep cleaning and exfoliating the skin. Some men shave daily while others shave at least twice a week.

STEP ONE: Find a cleanser for your skin that's not too soapy. Avoid products with a high alcohol content. Alcohol tends to dry the skin. A few of my favorite cleansers for morning and night are Aveeno Brightening Face Wash, Cetaphil Daily Cleanser or Granita Face Wash by Skintrium (mainly for problematic skin for men).

STEP TWO: Tone the skin. I'm not very big on toners unless they're organic or mild. The Calendula astringent by Kiehl's is great for all skin types. Kiehl's and Mario Badescu are great brands for all of your skincare needs.

STEP THREE: Find the perfect moisturizer with an SPF 30 or higher. You can also buy the SPF separately. If you have normal to dry, dry or combination skin, I'd suggest an all-in-one moisturizer from Kiehl's. Make sure the SPF is 30 or higher. I also love Cetaphil lotion for all skin types, including oily skin. You can have oily skin and still lack hydration. So, drinking loads of water daily is very helpful. Stay hydrated!

STEP FOUR: Use the above tips and remember if you're in the sun all day, SPF must be applied at least every 90 minutes or so. This is when the use of hats can be extremely useful. At the end of the day make sure you cleanse your skin. This removes free radicals and bacteria found in the environment. (Important for landscapers, construction workers or anyone working outdoors for long periods of time).

STEP FIVE: The above steps apply to men who shave or have beards. For conditioning beards, I suggest organic oils like sweet almond oil, lavender oil or organic coconut oil. These oils are all antibacterial and perfect to use after shaving. These oils also help with pre/post shave and can help prevent razor bumps. Rather than spending tons of money on designer shaving or beard products, invest in top grade organic oils that are a fraction of the cost.

I have been asked if men wear foundation, concealer, powder and bronzers. In my profession the answer is absolutely yes! The make-up is used in order to make talent (actors, models, singers) look more polished/refined. Some of my clients are pros and even know how they want it applied. There are so many new formulations in products on the market; all-in-one products are used for coverage to even out skin tone, as well as provide an instant tan, like tanning towels and sun protection. These products are sold in stores and spas around the globe. I have encountered men who use these items, which give a healthy and evened out glow to their skin.

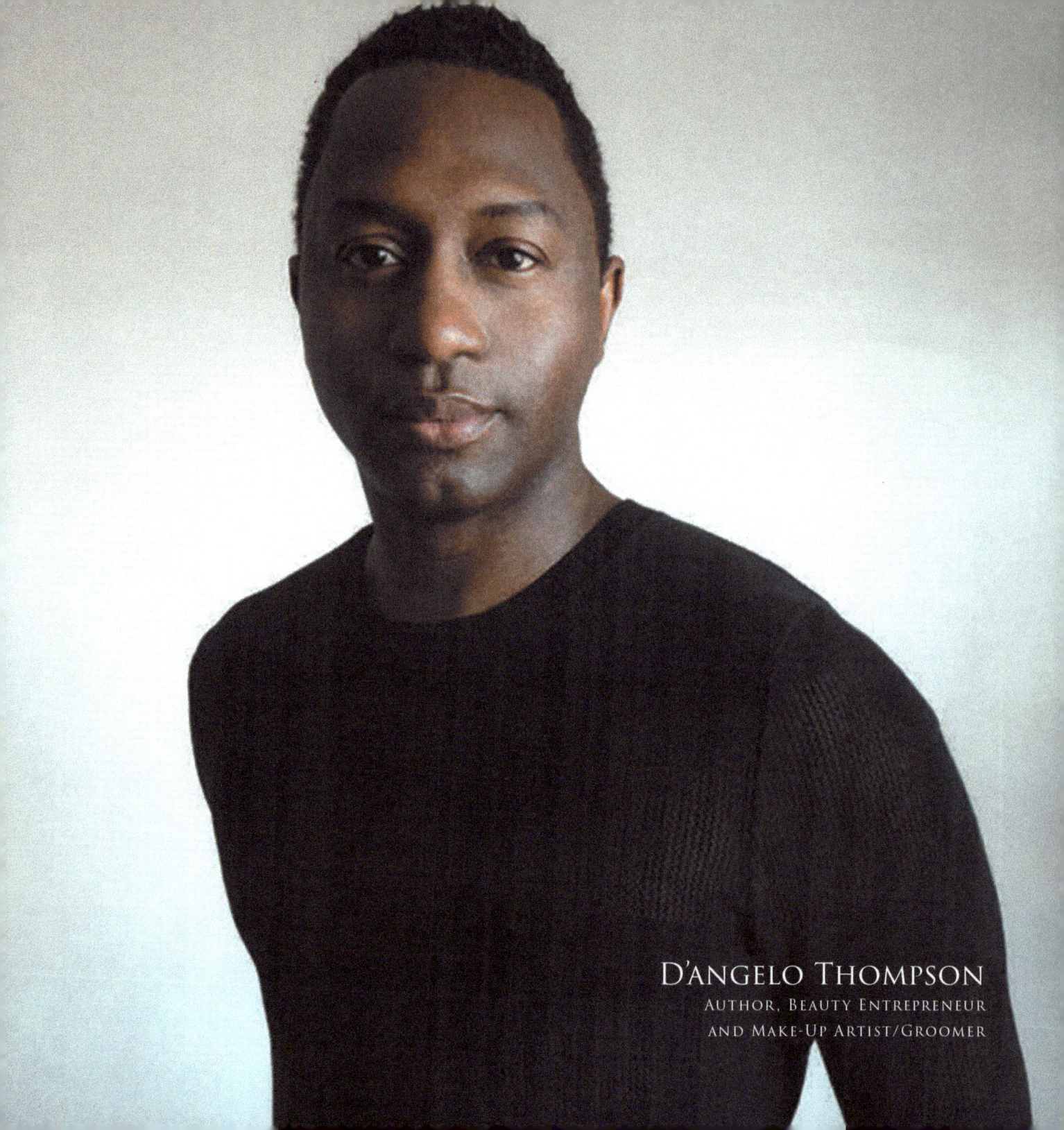

D'ANGELO THOMPSON
AUTHOR, BEAUTY ENTREPRENEUR
AND MAKE-UP ARTIST/GROOMER

Personal Experience

Through the years I have dealt with ingrown hairs and mild breakouts, so I was on a quest for the perfect shave. I wanted my skin to have that same glow and freshness that shows immediately after a shave. Like most teens, I was taught to use shaving cream and single blade razors purchased from the drug store or getting a shave at the barber shop with a straight razor. I learned pretty early on, due to my sensitive skin, neither worked for me and caused a massive breakout of ingrown hairs no matter what was recommended.

In my early twenties while working at Neiman Marcus in San Francisco, California, I graduated to using Aramis Lab Series Cooling Shaving Cream, which I used with two single-blade disposable razors. One razor for my neck and one razor for my face. I found using two razors gave me great results. In time, many razor manufacturers started to upgrade their blade qualities, which helped give me a better/closer shave. As we get older our skin texture changes, so I needed to change how I shaved. At that time I was introduced to shaving oils, triple blade razors and shaving creams by The Art of Shaving, which worked extremely well and caused minimal ingrown hairs.

However, I can honestly say that meeting dermatologist, Dr. Virgil Hatcher, New York City, changed my skin forever. Both celebrity men and women with whom I worked demanded to know how I was taking care of my skin. I had finally found my secret weapon.

CALL A DOCTOR

Dr. Virgil Hatcher of Chelsea Dermatology/Mount Sinai suggested I do blue laser hair removal because I always preferred to be clean shaven. After 12 or so painful procedures to remove my facial/beard hair (numbing cream is used), I had new skin and slower beard growth. I haven't used a razor in over 13+ years! I only use a depilatory cream by Magic Razorless Cream Shave, along with a warm and wet washcloth, in order to remove the cream/hair after a few minutes (4 minutes is suggested by Magic Razorless Cream Shave). This is ideal for men prone to ingrown hairs or breakouts after shaving. It's worth the cost and will save you money in the long run. Keep in mind, everyone's facial hair growth and patterns are different, and, thankfully, I explored and used many options on myself and clients. I can give you my personal and professional opinion, but you have to explore different options to get the perfect shave.

For other skin issues such as patchiness or dryness on the face or body, talk to a dermatologist/medical aesthetician. You might have psoriasis or eczema, which may be mild or advanced cases, but most doctors can identify the problem. They will either suggest dietary changes or prescribe a medication.

The above steps can vary according to your skin's specific needs or concerns. Some men are extremely lucky and only have to use electric razors with a little moisturizing with SPF daily and exfoliating on occasion. Whatever your skincare needs are, find a skincare regimen that caters to your individual concerns.

BODY CARE

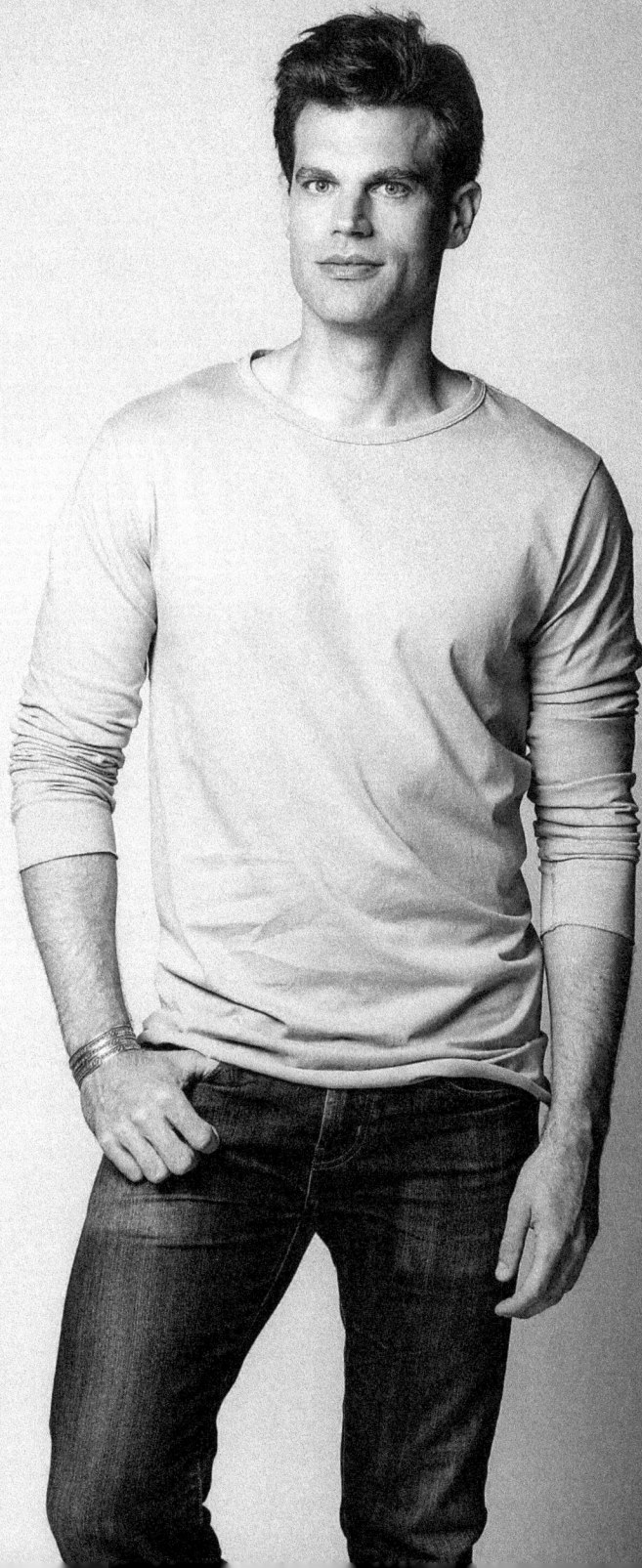

PAUL KOCH

PROJECT MANAGER / MODEL

Many experts say that hygiene is multifaceted. Diet, exercise and body care help to sustain good hygiene. Our cover model and professional project manager, Paul Koch, works hard at maintaining a healthy diet and fitness regimen.

I've always consulted with doctors and nutritionists when it comes to my diet, because everyone's nutritional and health needs are different. It is important to have an annual physical, which most of us avoid. You need to know what is going on with your temple.

Do research online about fitness or consult with a personal trainer and/or nutritionist in order to be better informed. You also have various books, videos and blogs about fitness online where you can tailor-make a regimen for the ideal body you want. I've also created an image board and have a screensaver of the male supermodel Chad White on my laptop, which helps me remain focused when I want to have that piece of cake or three slices of pizza (NOT!). An ideal diet, which is actually a lifestyle choice, is eating healthy and regularly working out your mind and body. This keeps you on the right track.

Body care is about being aware of your temple. Like every machine, it needs to be maintained and polished. Getting a haircut, manicure, pedicure and a shave are all forms self-care. It's not only to attract the opposite sex or partner.

A haircut or trim keeps your hair looking healthy. Using tons of hair products may leave the hair looking shiny or sculpted, but doesn't necessarily mean it's healthy. Celebrity hair stylist, Denine Smith of the Warren Tricomi Salon, NYC suggests to "never square up the nape of your neck, it looks dated and unattractive.

Also, avoid cookie cutter haircuts. You have to find what's ideal for your hair texture and lifestyle. Use shampoos and conditioners for your hair type, and use pomades and gels to control the hair or style. Don't overuse products." Many hairstylist suggest not shampooing everyday unless you're doing a hardcore workout routine.

Shaving is a daily process for most men, but the trend of the moment is having facial hair, which also must be maintained. (See the chapter on Skincare for maintaining facial hair.) It's best to trim your beard with shears or clippers and to use the same shampoo on your head as you do on your beard. Condition and moisturize your beard as suggested in the previous chapter by using organic oils, which are great and inexpensive alternatives.

STEP ONE: Other than showering twice daily, exfoliate the entire body at least twice a week. Exfoliation will slough off dead skin.

STEP TWO: Moisturize your skin after a shower or bathing, this helps to hydrate the skin. Some shower gels are 3-in-1 (cleanse, exfoliate, moisturize) and can be found at your local pharmacy or spa. If you have extra-dry skin, especially during the winter months, try heavy duty moisturizers. My favorite is Nivea 48-Hour Moisturizer for dry and extra-dry skin. I've been using Nivea religiously for over a decade, especially during the fall/winter months.

STEP THREE: At least once a month invest in having a manicure and pedicure. Not only is it good to maintain your nails, it is also very relaxing. Trust me, your wife, girlfriend or partner would agree.

MANSCAPING

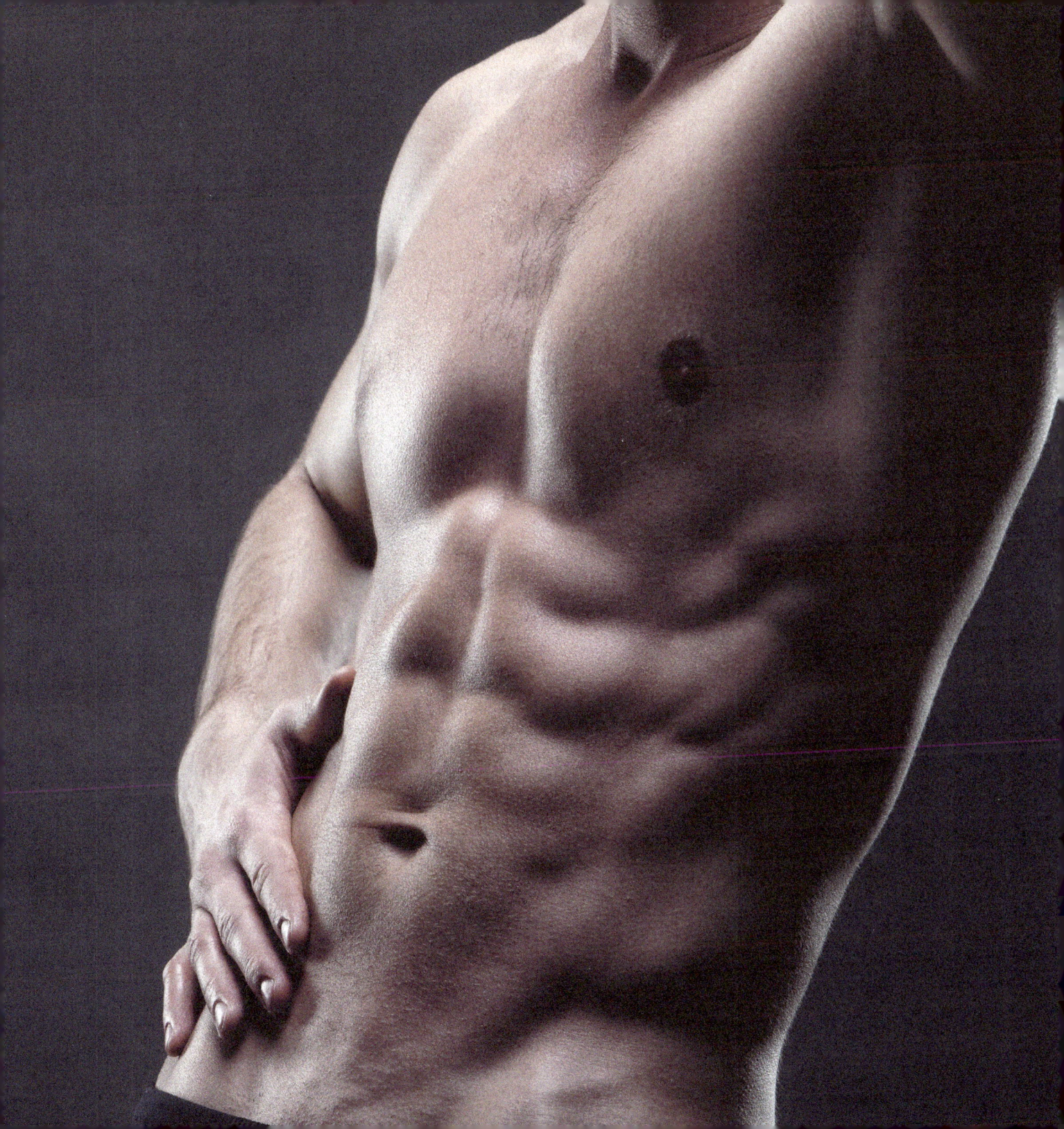

I highly advise doing a little manscaping at least every six weeks. You can do it at home if you don't feel comfortable having it done at a spa.

Simply trim down pubic hair with shears or clippers. Be extra careful around the testicles.

A lot of men like to have smooth chests and backs and there are many methods that work well for those areas. You could use a razor, but using clippers is the preferred method, as they cut down on ingrown hairs. You may opt to have a professional waxing as well. There are many do-it-yourself home kits and the most effective products include the hair removal with sugar or wax strips. This is, of course, a personal preference. A little manscaping is advised. My close female friends have shared with me that they appreciate a well-groomed man.

Body hair, or lack thereof, is not a bad or unmasculine thing. Hair helps to trap our body odor and to keep hygiene in check. Most women are attracted to the male pheromone, androstenol, which is a natural aphrodisiac. It typically comes out more in men when they sweat. All the more reason to work out and push harder at the gym!

I suggest every man experience a manicure and pedicure at least once in their lifetime, once a month is preferable. Manicures are great, especially if you work in construction or landscaping. A good manicure will eliminate the grime underneath the nails, which can be unhealthy for you and your partner. I will even go as far to say that dirty nails are noticed more times than not, especially on dates and in professional settings. In addition, taking care of your feet by having pedicures and moisturizing them is just as important as having well-manicured finger nails. No one wants to look at or feel gnarly feet in bed next to them.

On a daily basis we wash and moisturize our hands and bodies as needed even though our bodies produce natural oils, but sometimes, depending on which part of the world you live in or the season, your skin becomes dry and flaky. It's important to moisturize. Don't forget to moisturize the feet.

Something else that many women know that men do not, is the importance of exfoliating the body. There are many over the counter 2-in-1 or 3-in-1 body washes and scrubs on the market as stated in previous chapter. Exfoliating sloughs off dead skin and keeps the body looking and feeling invigorated. Exfoliating helps in blocking any skin irritations such as ingrown hairs, pimples and dry skin patches, especially on the back. There are many spas for men around the globe or you can go to a traditional Korean or Turkish bath for an inexpensive full body spa conditioning. I know many businessmen who swear by it. It's a great way to relax and release the stress we hold in our bodies.

Celebrity hairstylist, Denine Smith also suggest, "LUSH, a preservative-free line for the face and body". She and I are strong advocates for preservative-free and organic products for the skin, hair and body. LUSH, DoingLiving.com (Apothecary) and Whole Clarity are a few organic body brands on the market that I recommend. Take a little time to explore and research different products.

Avoid heavily perfumed products unless they include in their ingredients a natural scent such as lemongrass, lavender and sandalwood. Normally, heavily perfumed products are synthetic and are toxic to our bodies and the environment. It's important to be aware of these things even though I know it's easy to pick up something that is familiar to us. But, the more we know through science and research the more we understand about what we put in and on our bodies can be crucial to our long-term health.

ETHNIC SKIN

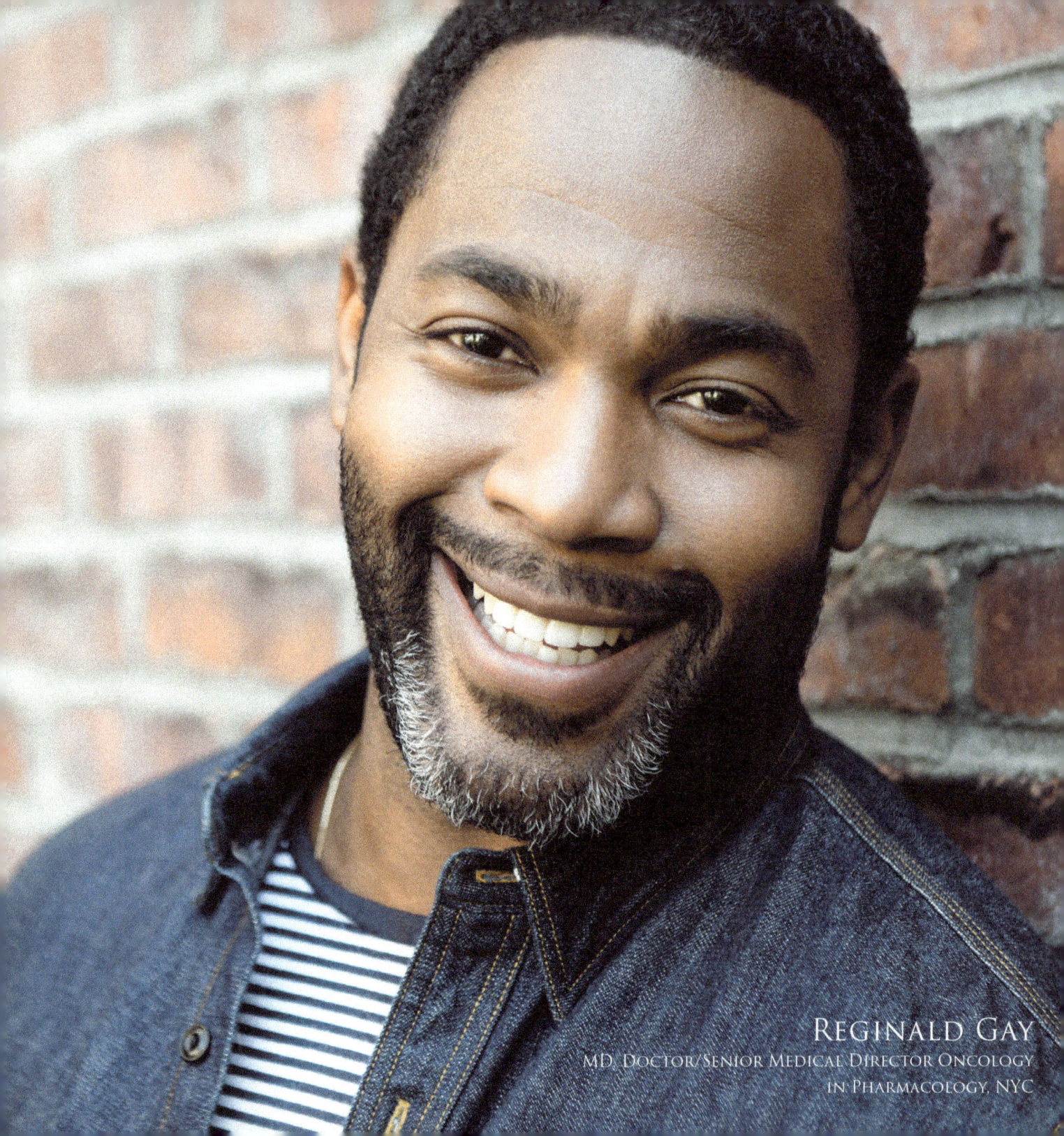

Reginald Gay
MD, Doctor/Senior Medical Director Oncology
in Pharmacology, NYC

As men of color, it is important to know what Dr. Reginald Gay, Dennis Howard (featured below) and I struggle with regarding our skin and hair, as well as what to be aware of when buying products. As discussed throughout the book, most of my suggestions apply to all men. I also want to discuss hyper pigmentation, dark spots and ingrown hairs, which also affect men of color more commonly.

Most men, especially men of color, think SPF is not important...this is a myth. We can get sunburned, have allergies to the sun or get diagnosed with skin cancer just as easily as men with a lighter skin shade. According to the Skin Cancer Foundation, "anyone can get skin cancer". Understand that moisturizing is equally as important as wearing sunscreen daily. The American Academy of Dermatology recommends applying a sunscreen with at least an SPF (Sun Protection Factor) of 30 and to reapply the sunscreen after 90 minutes if outdoors.

Sunscreen will also help with uneven skin tones, but there are also great over the counter creams to use in conjunction with moisturizer and sunscreen. Facial creams with Alpha Hydroxy Acids (Walgreen's Brand) or Salicylic Acid (Aveeno) will help with uneven skin tones. Also, Vitamin C serums and creams are effective as well and can be found in many cosmetic/skincare brands. These products may also be available at the office of a dermatologist or esthetician/facialist, which will offer stronger formulations. These creams and serums must be applied daily with a sunscreen to be effective. Higher concentrations of AHA, Salicylic Acid or Vitamin C, which work more rapidly, can be found at a licensed dermatologist. Other options to consider are retinol and laser skin treatments. It's imperative that you seek out a professional who understands the science behind darker skin tones/textures.

There are more aggressive skincare treatments that can be discussed with a licensed professional, such as laser treatments or bleaching creams. I had a laser treatment done to prevent ingrown hairs and hyper pigmentation over a decade ago and I still get compliments on my skin today.

Laser is not for everyone, so you must be diligent about selecting a licensed professional, as well as someone who understands and specializes in darker skin tones, as suggested by my New York based dermatologist Dr. Virgil Hatcher. There are many great dermatologist throughout the world, just ask for referrals. Word of mouth can be very useful!

Hyperpigmentation can be genetic, caused by high exposure to sun or skin damage linked to acne vulgaris. It can be treated by skin bleaching treatments, Retin-A or Alpha Hydroxy creams. You must be persistent in treating it daily. Sun protection is essential. If not treated properly it can become more problematic.

Ingrown hairs can occur after shaving the face, head or body. There are many ways to avoid ingrown hairs as suggested by NYC based barber, David Rakhminov. Rakhminov suggests "using a warm cloth before shaving, apply shaving gel or cream, using a straight razor or high-end disposable razor, rinse and apply a warm towel again. Use a firming mask post shave and moisturizer afterwards." The Art of Shaving suggests a similar procedure by "using a warm cloth, then shaving oil by massaging it in in order to lift hairs, apply shaving cream with a shaving brush and then use a razor. After shaving use a post shave moisturizer that's enriched with natural oils for restoring the skin." All of these methods worked for me when I use to shave. I've only used a disposable or electric razor in the past 10+ years, if there was an emergency. After I had my laser treatment over a decade ago, I've only had to use a depilatory, Magic Razorless Cream Shave in Regular on my beard area for 3 to 5 minutes. Afterwards, I apply organic coconut oil, which I infuse with organic lavender oil or sweet almond oil, all over my face. This keeps my skin youthful, as the oils are naturally antibacterial and help combat any ingrown hairs.

Men have a plethora of options from which to choose in order to achieve a clean shave. Make sure your barber or hairstylist cleans/disinfects their tools. This will also help with a perfect shave, as well as avoid any other skin rashes or irritations. I've seen horrific skin abrasions and scarring from unsanitary hair tools. Be certain your personal tools at home are also sharp and clean.

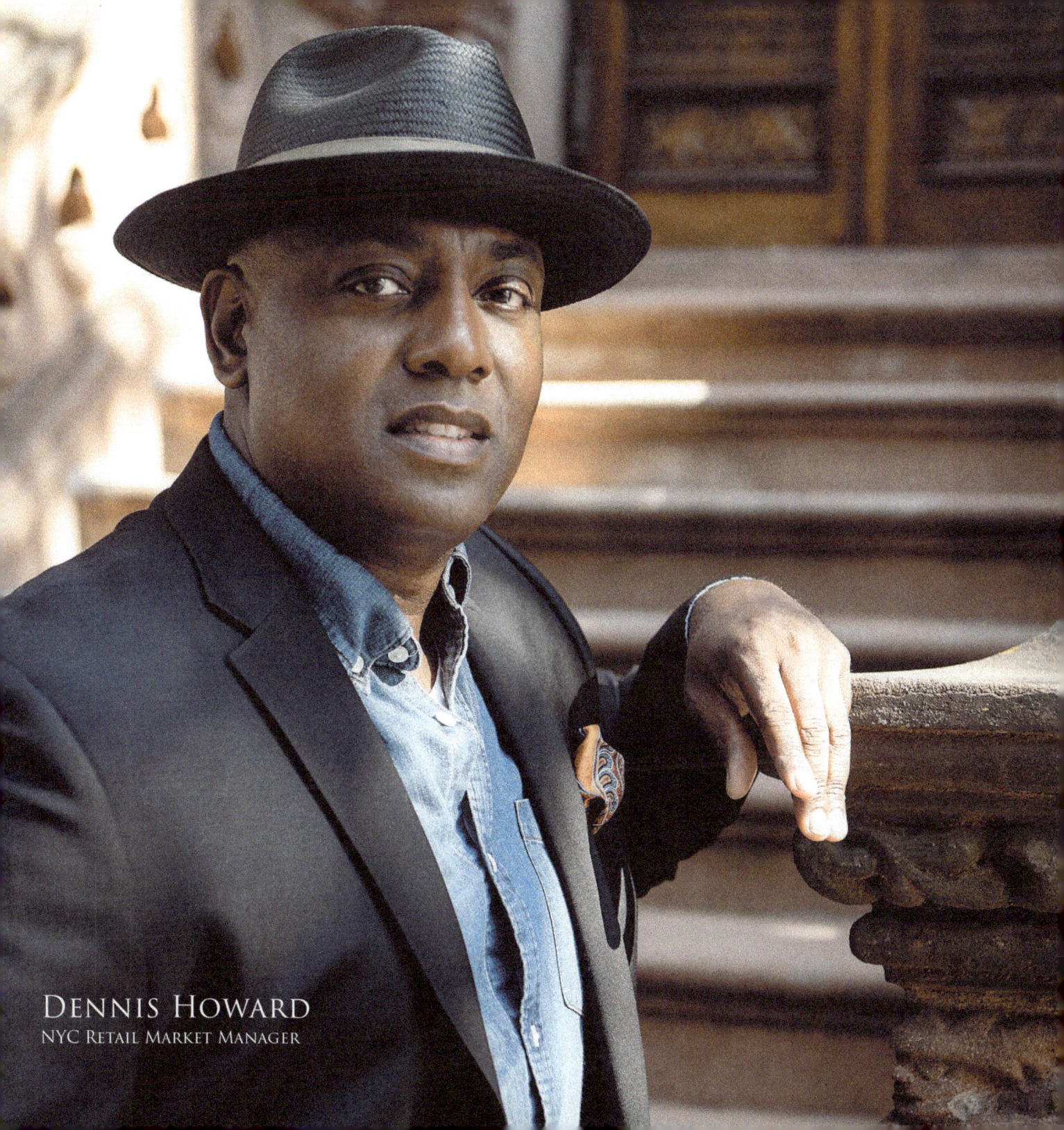

DENNIS HOWARD
NYC Retail Market Manager

HAIR

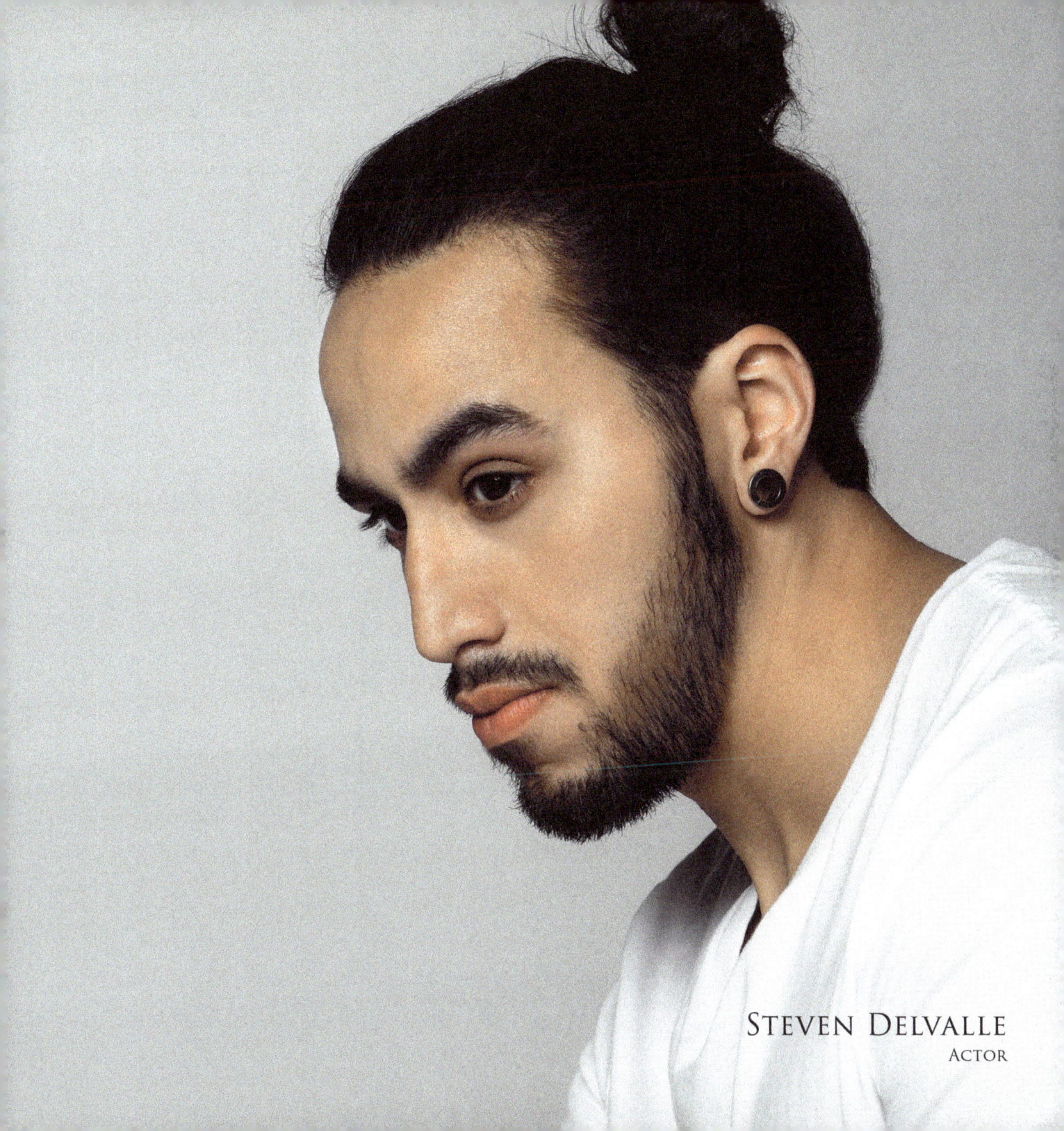

STEVEN DELVALLE
ACTOR

Hair care is important whether you have a buzz cut, low Ceasar, a trendy swoop or hipster top knot, like the image above of Steven DelValle. Great hair is hair that is well conditioned, smells great and is trimmed regularly. In other words, hair has to be healthy!

Just as there have been advancements in skin and body care products, there have been massive improvements in hair care for men. Products such as vitamin enriched, paraben-free, naturally sourced shampoos and conditioners, hair loss prevention shampoos like Rogaine, Nioxin, Biotin or Q10 and vitamins, can all be found over the counter. Look for product lines like Aveda, Bumble and Bumble, IGK, Kiehls, Oribe, as well as organic vegan brands like Yarok, which are all innovative products and provide a progressive approach to haircare. Many of these hair product lines also cater to longer hair, color treated hair and even beards. There are products available that will suit all of your needs and concerns. Be certain to talk to the professionals, sample products and ask questions when it comes to grooming and hair styling.

I chatted with a few hair stylists and brand ambassadors for this book and all agreed it is best to get a haircut that is suited for your hair and texture. Try not to overuse styling products and avoid products heavy in alcohol. "Take it easy on the hair gel fellas", advises both David Rakman (Barber) and Denine Smith (Hair Stylist).

Most men I know are very particular about how their hair is cut, be it with clippers, razors or with sheers. Due to their demanding lifestyles and schedules, the cut must look great when it's initially done and when it grows out. Even with a hectic schedule, I manage to visit the barber once a week. When I wore longer, trendier hairstyle's years ago, I would frequent the salon stylist every two weeks for the Japanese precision cut done with shears.

Many exclusive men's spas are popping up in cities throughout   the world, which cater to the art of shaving, facials, beard trimming and upkeep, as well as scissor and razor cuts, barbering, shoe shine, dry cleaning, manicures and pedicures. These spas for men offer a full-service experience. What a genius idea!

Men are no strangers to coloring their hair, but most choose colors that are too dark and look unnatural, especially as they age. As suggested to women, choose colors that are softer around the face and add dimension. This is true for any shade, whether it's black, dark brown, auburn, red, blonde or platinum. "Often times men get stuck using the same hair color as women, which isn't ideal being that most men have ash/cool tones in their hair. Now brands are starting to cater and create color lines devoted to men", says hair colorist Marco Guglielmino of Marco NYC Salon.

Currently, there are trendy and bold colors for the hair that are semi-permanent. Have fun with these colors! Creatives do. Hair color is all about preference, but acquire knowledge about hair coloring when making choices about your appearance.

When choosing the right color be careful not to over process or damage the hair. Seek out hair color that has built-in moisturizing and nourishing qualities, like organic hair color at selective salons and brands like Garnier, Just For Men and others that you can purchase over the counter.

Gray or salt & pepper natural hair color can be amazing and I believe men get better and more distinguished as we age. Look at the talented and handsome icons such as Morgan Freeman, George Clooney and Anderson Cooper. Don't be afraid to rock silver hair. There's nothing better than a person accepting and aging gracefully. Part of the aging process may include losing hair and having a thinning hairline. When this happens, opt for shorter precision cuts. If you're in the public eye there are products that fill in bald spots or thinning hair (Toppik--microfibers are used to mimic hair), as well as lines of sprays or waxes to fill in bald spots and remove the shine. I utilize these assortment of products often on set. The effect looks natural and is excellent for photo shoots, in-person meetings and on camera. Try professional or theatrical make-up shops for these specific products like Alcone, Cinema Secrets and Amazon (all online or a phone call away).

Denine Smith suggests, "for more curly or kinky textured hair, it's important to get trims regularly-- every 6 to 8 weeks. Avoiding regular trims can cause split ends and/or hair breakage." If you use texturizing products and hair color, I would suggest seeing your stylist every two weeks for either a deep conditioning or trim. This will maintain healthy looking hair."

Here are a few firm do's and don't's:

> Do use sulfate-free and paraben-free shampoos.

> Do use rich conditioners & masks that make hair more supple, manageable and tangle free.

> Do use hydrating finishing creams and oils, which leave a lasting shine.

> Do properly shampoo and condition your hair at least twice a week to avoid itchiness or scalp issues.

> Don't use excessive heat.

> Don't wear tight hairstyles, which can weaken the follicle and cause hair loss.

The above mentioned hair rules can be applied to both men and women, but I stress it more with men because self-care is not always at the top of our priority list, either due to exhaustion or lack of knowledge.

STEP ONE: Shampoo hair at least twice a week as suggested by many hair professionals. Condition hair every other week and at least once a week if you have a drier scalp. Use sulfate-/paraben-free shampoos and conditioners.

STEP TWO: Avoid overusing hair gels, creams and products with alcohol. Use hydrating creams to style hair while wet or dry.

STEP THREE: Get hair trimmed regularly, at least every 6 to 8 weeks to avoid breakage or split ends.

STEP FOUR: If you choose to color, straighten or texturize hair, trim and deep condition every 4 to 6 weeks. I would also suggest doing natural oil treatments that you can do at home or at renowned organic hair salons like YAROK in New York City.

STEP FIVE: Be faithful to the hairstylist or barber you trust. They understand your hair and hopefully will keep it healthy.

~

If you choose to let your hair grey naturally, follow the above rules and be certain when using hair styling products to avoid products with color. This can cause the hair to look dull and tint the brilliance of the grey hair.

~

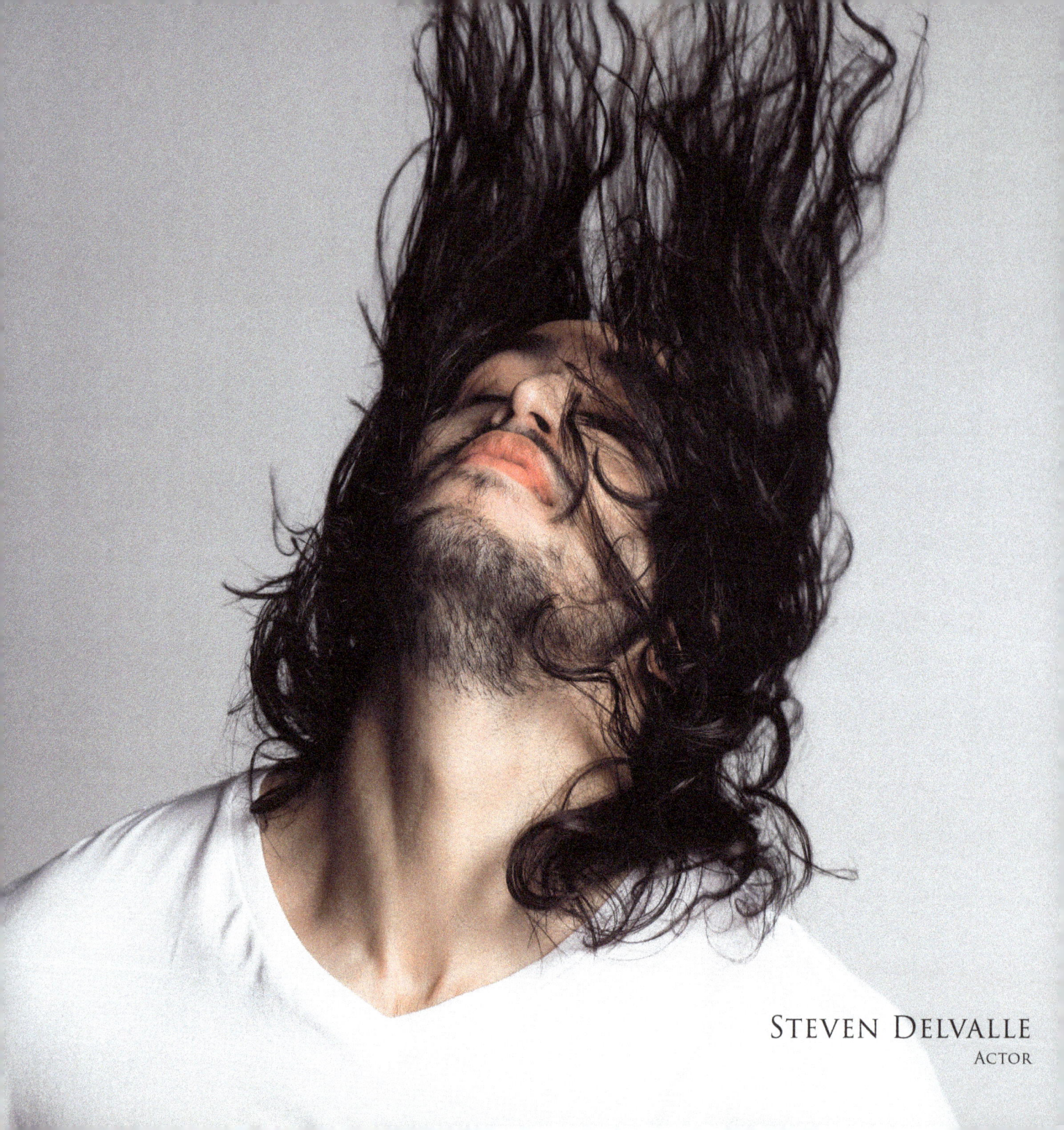

STEVEN DELVALLE
ACTOR

AGING

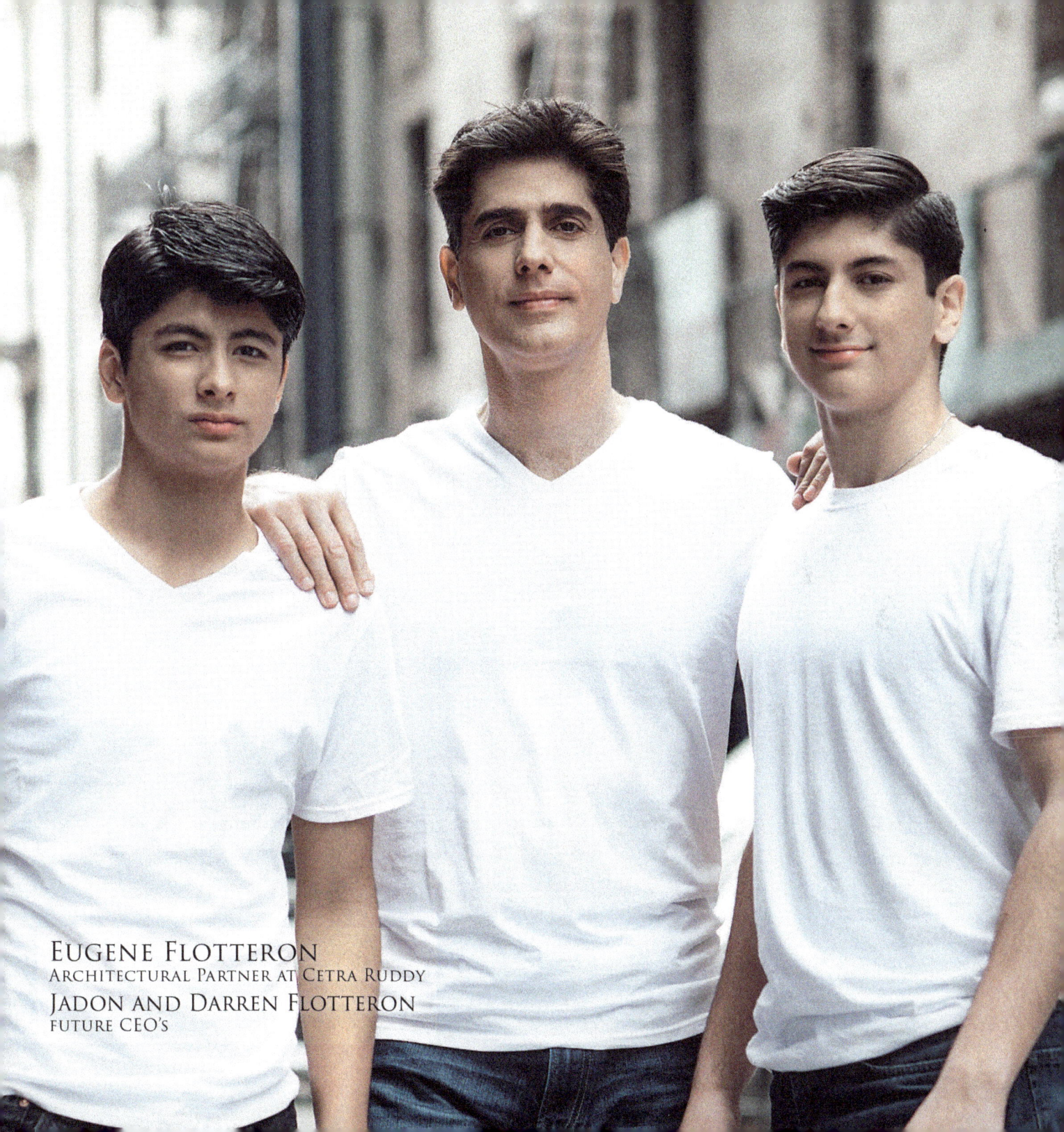

EUGENE FLOTTERON
ARCHITECTURAL PARTNER AT CETRA RUDDY

JADON AND DARREN FLOTTERON
FUTURE CEO's

Getting older can be difficult for some, but I think "age is a privilege", which was a hashtag at a friend's 50th birthday party. The words reminded me of how precious life is. Men and women get better with age, they become more solid with who they are and strong in their wisdom, like my dear friend above with his sons, Eugene Flotteron. Self-confidence comes with age and it's intoxicatingly sexy.

Throughout the book, I talked about self-care; this doesn't stop as you get older. There's nothing more alluring than a well-dressed, polished man of a certain age. Taking the time to groom and taking care of yourself-mentally and physically-is important at any age. Many health professionals state that as we age we need to exercise regularly; not only to keep the heart healthy, but to radiate healthiness from the inside out. Healthy eating, taking supplements and sustaining a solid fitness routine are daily practices which help in the aging process.

There are certain foods we must avoid according to MensHealth.com There are leading doctors who stress that eating these foods can be linked to many health issues, as well as breast cancer in men and low testosterone levels. Your best option is to consult with your doctor and nutritionist. They will provide the most up-to-date information. Most professionals will tell you to eat organic foods, drink leafy green juices, as well as other fruit and vegetables, as the best way to have optimal health.

Life is about reinvention and evolving. We never stop learning. Since we know that, make sure you stay abreast on newer ways to stay healthy. Always avoid food trends and focus on what's healthiest for your body type and lifestyle. Sometimes it's something as simple as a refresher in your wardrobe, a shift in your color palette or a new style of clothing. There are many male and female stylists and wardrobe consultants at department stores, showrooms, high-end boutiques or freelancers that can fine tune your look. Take the time to invest in yourself. This not only helps you feel good, but look good as well. It's called "retail therapy" for a reason.

Not only is eating healthy and regular exercise beneficial to you, it also helps combat depression, according to the National Institute of Mental Health. NIMH states that "men handle depression differently than women." Depression can be triggered by stress in the workplace, hormones or genetics. It's typically a combination of all three. So, when you go for a physical always consider your mental health as well. The reason I wanted to assert this in my book on Men's Grooming is because men are more likely to commit suicide than women, according to many studies.

It's not only about the outer appearance for me, but how a man feels mentally as well. Sadly, I've known young men who have taken their own lives in their late 20's to early 30's. It's important to talk to someone. The National Suicide Prevention Hotline is 1-800-273-8255 (US Only). The calls remain anonymous. However, if you are in a serious crisis please call 911 first.

Routine is important, but it's also great to shift from the same routine to another one in order for your body and mind to expand. Similar to many sports, you can't always play the same plays, you have to switch it up, which builds your strength and endurance. Also, your adversary won't know what to expect. This ensures a win. In life, we have to switch it up sometimes. I was always an active child. I played most sports, but I was not very good at basketball. Unfortunately, I didn't get that gene from my parents. As I got older I was drawn more to the arts. Ironically, as I get older I appreciate more competitive sports and enjoy watching tennis, volleyball and soccer. A peaceful activity for me is running. I practice yoga in order to relieve stress. Participating in group sports, a solitary workout or a good jog surrounded by nature are ways to stay focused/centered in your everyday life. In the midst of our busy lives, please take the time to explore nature, travel and try new things outside of your comfort zone. I promise you will find magic in those moments.

In all stages of life it's about self-care and finding a zen place in all moments. As we get older we gain wisdom if we embrace the lessons life presents to us. All of the men whom I've encountered throughout the years, who have taken care of themselves, actually have gotten better looking as they have aged and have become more confident with their style choices.

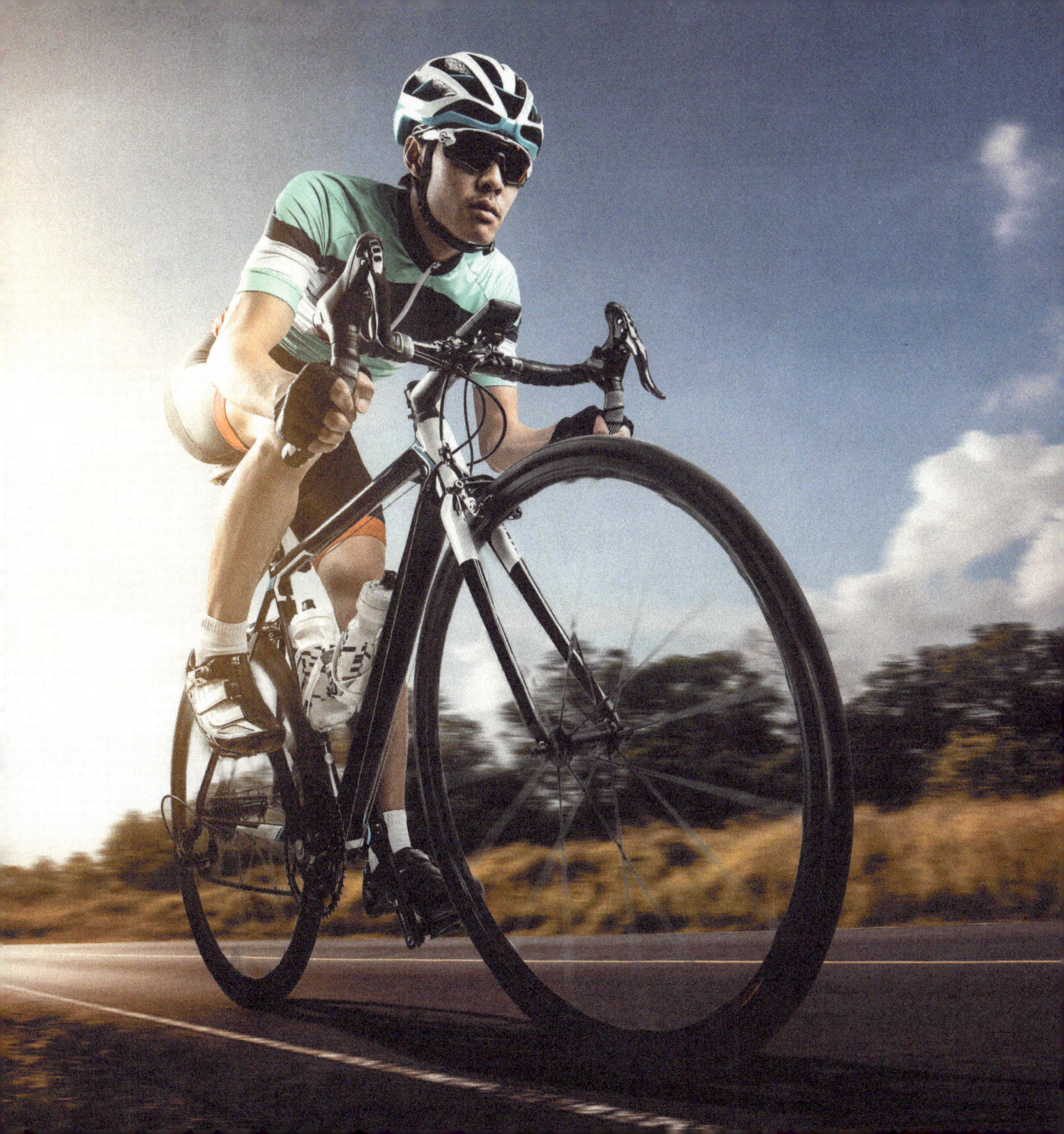

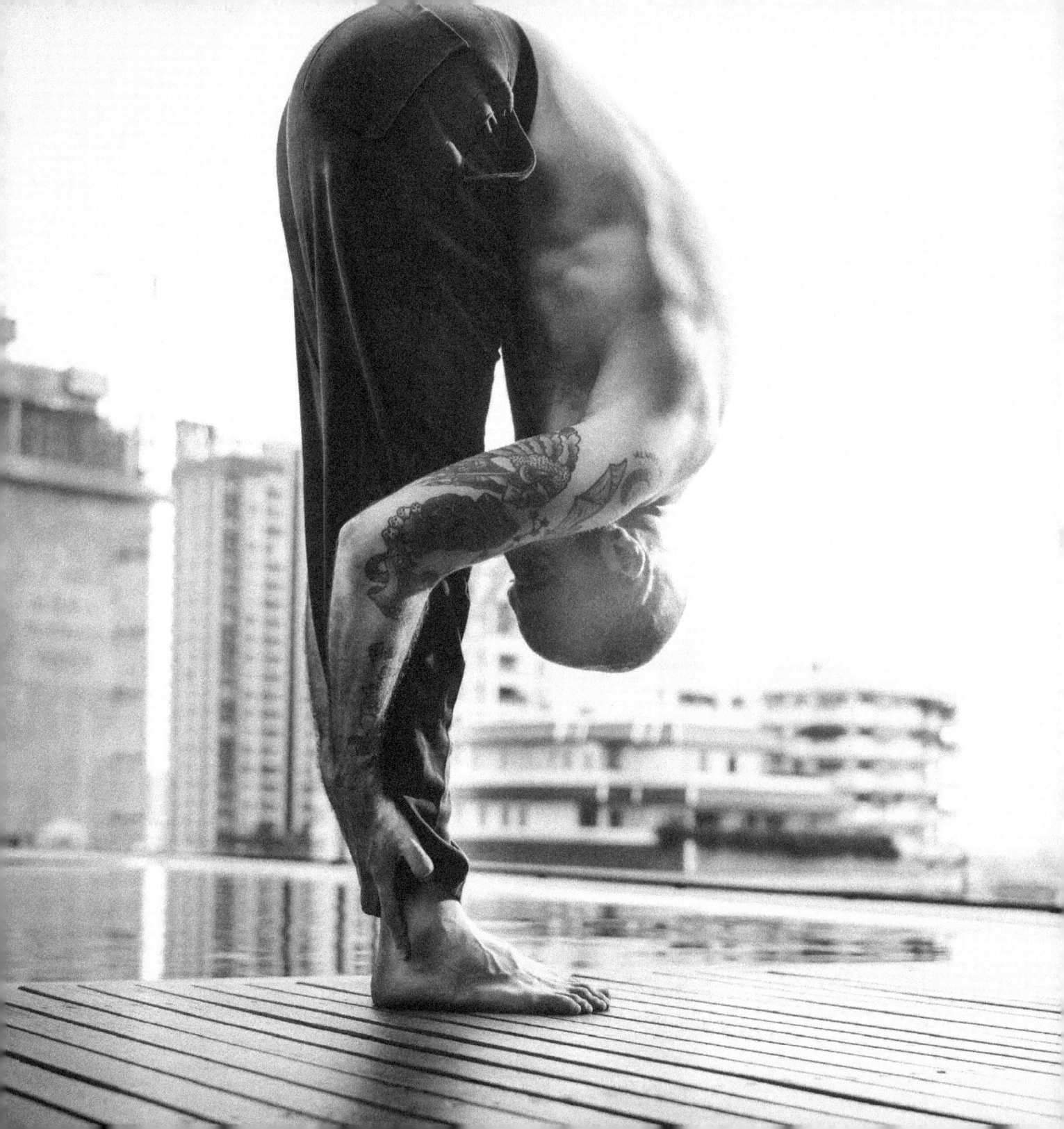

HEALTH + FITNESS

It's important for men to remain in tune with our bodies and stay on top of our health concerns and needs. So often we see the doctor when things have escalated. It saddens me most when we hear about dear friends or family members dying young from illnesses that could have been prevented. Early detection and treatment could help save a life.

It can slip our minds easily, but it's so important to have an annual physical and get blood work done. I hate the blood work part, but it's necessary. I suggest getting a yearly physical around the time of your birth date. I do this yearly. It's helped me maintain a healthy and well-balanced life.

According to the CDC, the top two causes of death in men are heart disease and cancer, which are preventable with early detection and annual physicals. Of course, genetics, diet and exercise factor into our optimal health as well. As long as we are proactive participants in the process of great nutrition, exercise and having a positive mindset, it's the best we can do for ourselves.

You may ask, what does my health have to do with grooming? Your hair, skin and overall body health are connected. Treat them like the Holy Trinity. Healthiness comes from the inside out. Mental health is definitely one part of the whole picture. I remember years ago working with a very polished and handsome journalist. On the outside he looked great, like a sculpted Versace model, but the more I interacted with him, I saw his skin smothered with foundation and bronzer and his hair was heavily gelled. His oral hygiene was lacking as well, it was clear that there was a deeper health issue going on with him.

We get stuck playing these masculine roles assigned to us by society, which inevitably cut our life span down 10-20 years. The average woman lives 5-10 years longer than her spouse. I've observed women outliving their male partners by 20 years. So, I will talk about this until I'm blue in the face; men should take responsibility for their own health and well-being.

During the months of January and February of 2017, I was feeling fatigued. I couldn't sleep and felt depressed. I thought it was just seasonal mood disorder, which most people who live in the Northeast and Northwest of North America suffer from seasonally. I decided to get my yearly physical a month or so early. Thankfully, everything was great except that my Vitamin D levels were tremendously low. This explained it all. Despite my regular exercise and eating healthy, I was lacking something we all need--sun! The sun provides us with Vitamin D. It is our major source of it. I ended up taking Vitamin D twice daily. Without a daily dose of the sun my entire life was thrown off balance.

Even though I've chatted about and suggested products for skin and hair, it's also a great idea to take a break and allow the body and skin to take care of themselves. I call these "detox days". You would use only the products absolutely necessary and leave the rest in the medicine cabinet. I find this is helpful when you get breakouts or have hair issues. By the process of elimination you can determine what really works or doesn't.

Like most, men are influenced by advertising and social media, but you must remember, not one formula works for all men, as I have discussed in this book. Explore different options, educate yourselves and talk to professionals about what could work best for you. Even with that knowledge, sometimes you just have to switch it up. Also, be mindful of the expiration dates of products. Please throw them out once they have expired.

SEEK OUT A MENTOR

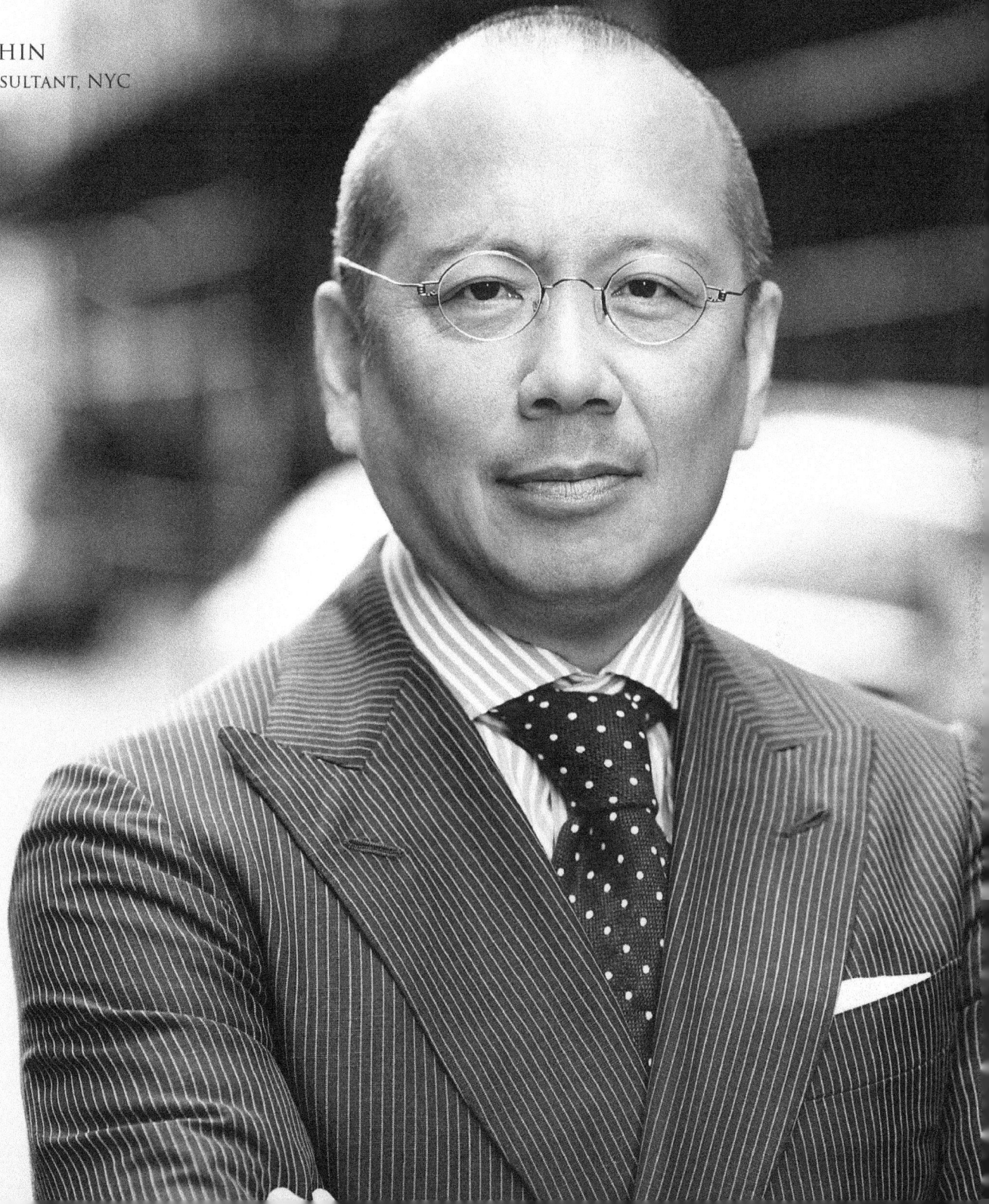

The stylish man on the previous page (who is also my friend) is someone I consider a mentor both personally and professionally, especially when it comes to style. David Chin flies under the radar, but styles some of the most talented, celebrated and powerful men in the world. Yet, he maintains balance within his personal life as a dad and professional life as a jet-setting go-to fashion influencer.

You may have had a mentor throughout your education, on the job, or with building your finances/wealth. It is important to seek out mentors when it comes to your style, over all aesthetic, learning new grooming tips or a fitness regimen. Don't be afraid to ask questions. Having a mentor is another way of fine-tuning your highest possible self.

At every age, I've been able to gauge when someone really had my back or was just giving me lip service. The person in your life that gives you the most honest, respectful and loving advice is someone to listen to or at least consider what they're saying. Sometimes when it comes from family or your significant other, we have a tendency to tune them out. I've been guilty of this as well. But, hidden beneath that "nagging" is a sincere concern for your well-being. It's how you choose to receive the information and observations given to you.

Some men prefer a coach's approach, which is stereotypically an approach of no-nonsense. Use whatever works best for you. Use that to propel your goals to the next level.

One of the most essential tools we have as we grow and evolve are accountability partners. A person who genuinely will make you affirm and follow through on your promises to yourself and others. Whether you are choosing a trainer, barber, hairstylist, nutritionist or guru, you need that person to give it to you straight. This practice has helped me grow the most as a man, artist and entrepreneur.

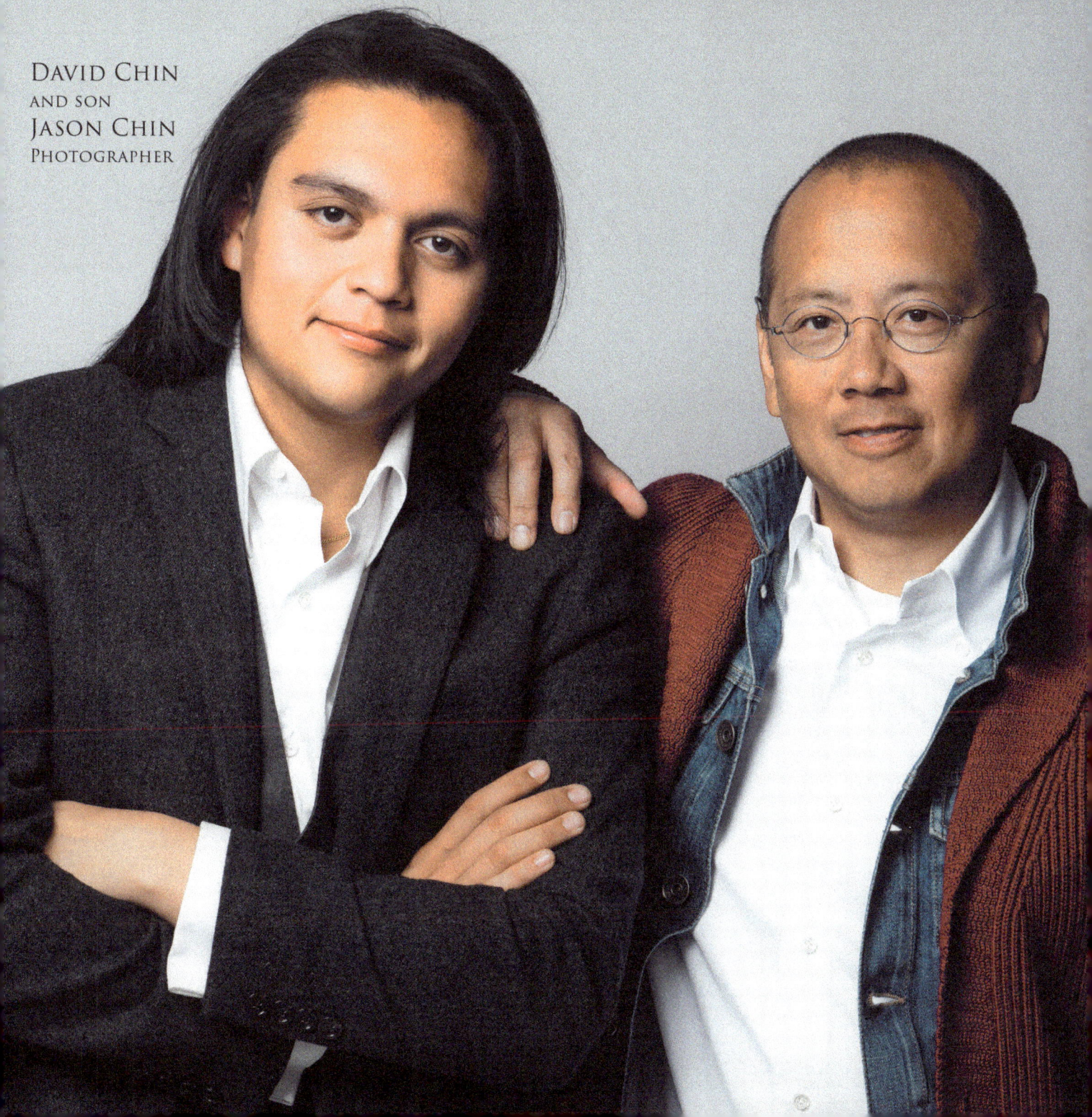

DAVID CHIN
AND SON
JASON CHIN
PHOTOGRAPHER

MEN'S GROOMING

This men's grooming book is more about personal care and is intended to give you useful information for your day-to-day lives, as well as inspire you to get up and move, inspire others, mentor, be mentored, volunteer and take care of yourself and loved ones!

As we evolve with our personal grooming, let's elevate the mind, body and soul. All else will align...I promise.

The image above of David Chin and his son, Jason Chin, illustrates that we receive many cues from our parents/guardians, and especially our fathers when we are young men.

TO MY READERS A SPECIAL THANK YOU
FOR TAKING THIS JOURNEY WITH ME
INTO THE ART OF MEN'S GROOMING,
WHICH IS BOOK NUMBER THREE OF
THE ENHANCED BEAUTY SERIES. I HOPE
THAT I HAVE PROVIDED ENOUGH
INFORMATION AND TIPS FOR YOU TO
USE. IT IS MY PLEASURE FOR YOU TO
SHARE THE INFORMATION PROVIDED IN
THIS BOOK WITH YOUR FATHER,
BROTHER, SON, FRIEND, COLLEAGUE, OR
PARTNER IN YOUR LIFE. THEY WILL
HAVE THE TOOLS NEEDED TO LOOK
THEIR ABSOLUTE BEST AND BEYOND.

BE THE GIANT YOU WERE BORN TO BE.

XOXO
D'ANGELO

Enhanced *Beauty*

MEN'S GROOMING

Enhanced *Beauty*

MEN'S GROOMING

*by Daytime Emmy Award Winning
Hairstylist and Nominated Make-Up Artist*

D'ANGELO THOMPSON

CPSIA information can be obtained
at www.ICGtesting.com
Printed in the USA
LVHW070048110219
607037LV00048B/474/P

9 781546 265832